CW00767072

QUICKIES

QUIVER

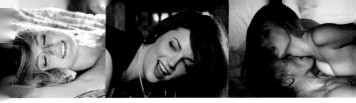

Contents

1. The Morning Horn
2. Happy Birthday
3. Wake Her Up with Lovers' T
4. Wake Him Up with Teabagging
5. Alarm Call
6. Making Juice
7. A Pair of Fried Eggs
8. Breakfast Buns
9. Pain Au Chocolat
10. Morning Breathless
11. Cutting It Close
12. Showered with Affection
13. Diet Cock Break
14. Box Lunch
15. Toss His Salad
16. Stuffed Sandwich
17. Ass-Kissing Lunch
18. 12 O' Cock
19. Eating In
20. Finger Sandwich
21. Tied-Up Afternoon
22. Afternoon Delight
23. Sneaky Sandwich
24. Lunchtime Liaison
25. Take Dicktation
26. Wash and Go
27. Naked Lunch
28. Lazy Lunch
29. A Filling Lunch
30. Bathroom Bliss
31. Silent Night
32. Vampire Kisses
33. In for the Night
34. Dirty Dancing
35. Stress Release
36. Prostate with Pleasure
37. Bath then Bed
38. Sleeping Like a Log
39. Stroke of Midnight
40. Sweet Dreams
41. One Night in Bangkok
42. Cocktail Time
43. Window (Un)Dressing
44. Rock-a-Bye-Baby
45. Open Wide
46. CAT Nap
47. Bedtime Buddies
48. Pillow Talk

How to Use This Book

Nowadays, we live increasingly busy lives. For too many of us, time is short, expectations are high, and pressure is everywhere. Often, in the struggle to fit everything in, it's sex that falls between the cracks. Before long, "Not tonight, dear," can turn into "When did we last get it on?" and it can be all too easy to find yourself gradually falling into the dreaded rut. But there's no need for your sex life to suffer simply because you've got so much else to fit into your day.

If you want to have great sex, you need to prioritize it, and that means making time for it. However, that doesn't mean you need to find an extra day in the week or even extra hours in the day. Instead, by embracing quickies as part of your love life, you can enjoy a sexy "snack" that can help keep your hunger sated until you have time to settle down for a proper feed. Heck, you might even decide that you'd rather have a handful of snacks than a three course meal.

Fast sex doesn't have to mean unsatisfying sex. Although the word "quickies" may conjure up hard and fast passion, that's only one way to get your rocks off in record time. Choosing a position that allows for lots of clitoral stimulation, rocking rather than thrusting, or adding a helping hand are just a few of the things that can help speed a woman's orgasm. And if it's the man who tends to be the longer-lasting partner, lube, prostate stimulation and throwing in some sexy visuals for good measure can all help put a rocket up his—err—rocket.

That's before you even take into account that sex isn't just about inserting a penis into a vagina. Your hands, mouth, and indeed, almost every inch of your body can be used for sexual satisfaction, whether your own, your partner's, or better yet, both.

We're also lucky enough to live in a time when toys and erotic novelties of all varieties abound, designed with both male and female sexual pleasure in mind. They are perfect for when your spirit is willing but flesh is weak and ideal if you want to stimulate maximum erogenous zones in minimum time.

Of course, quickies don't always have to involve mutual climax. There's nothing wrong with pleasuring your partner and letting him or her return the favor at a later point, as long as you're both happy with it. A swift but focused oral session in the morning when your lover's got limited time but really wants to come could well serve as mental foreplay to keep your mind on sex all day. With any luck, when your lover gets home, he or she will be eager to return the favor; whether with a reciprocal quickie or a more extended session depends on how much time you have to play with.

This book will provide you with forty-eight quick and easy ways to get intimate no matter what time it is. Too tired for sex when you finally get to bed? Try getting it on in the morning instead. Hate mornings with a passion? Have a lunchtime treat that really will leave you feeling satisfied all afternoon. Changing the time of day that you have sex, along with the positions and techniques that you use, can help reinvigorate your love life and keep things fresh too.

From oral sex techniques to manual mastery, toy tricks to positions, everything in the book can be done in under twenty minutes (though a few techniques do require a little preparation). And if you have any extra time to spare, what better way to make the most of it than with more romping?

The techniques in this book are just a few of the ways in which you can enjoy fast sex with your lover. Rather than offering a rigid list of things to do, they offer a smorgasbord of suggestions for ways to speed things along during sex. If you don't like the exact details of any of the suggestions, change the things you don't like and add some things that you do. And if you know there's a certain technique that is sure to get your lover off in record time, incorporate it into your sex play.

Much as a good recipe book offers a selection of easily adapted base dishes, allowing you scope to play with the exact flavors yourself, this book presents a number of core concepts that can be tailored to suit your desires (and indeed, your gender preference and sexuality).

If you want to get playful and start creating your own quickie moves, the following lists may help. Simply choose the attributes that you want in sex to help both of you get off, and combine the various sex acts in whichever way most appeals. Simply discussing which acts and positions appeal and which leave you cold should help you both get to know each other much more intimately, which can also lead to better sex.

GREAT POSITIONS FOR CLITORAL STIMULATION

CAT (Coital Alignment Technique)
The man penetrates the woman missionary style then moves so that his pelvis is above her and lies flat on top of her. The woman then grinds her clitoris against the base of the man's shaft. As the position is more focused on clitoral stimulation than thrusting, the man may need to start thrusting once the woman has reached climax.

Cowgirl
The man lies on his back and the woman straddles him, facing him. This allows lots of scope for kissing, and the more a woman leans forward, the greater amount of clitoral stimulation she can get. This is a great position for first-time strap-on sex, too, as the receiving partner can control the depth of penetration.

Scissoring
Both partners lie facing each other and the woman slides one of her thighs between her partner's. Her partner penetrates her, and the woman rocks and grinds against the thigh while her partner thrusts. This position can also be used for anal sex but can be tricky to get into.

GREAT POSITIONS FOR DEEP PENETRATION

Doggie Style
The woman kneels on all fours in front of the man. For strap-on sex, this position is reversed.

Standing Sex
The woman leans against the wall and bends over from the waist to deepen penetration. Again, this position can be reversed for strap-on sex.

Raised Missionary
The woman lies on her back with a pillow underneath her hips. Her partner penetrates from above, supporting his weight on his arms. This variation of missionary can also work with strap-on sex. Some believe the muscles relax more in missionary position, making it a more comfortable position for the person receiving anal sex. However, it can be a little tricky to get into position for anal play, so you may find it easier once anal sex is something you're already familiar with doing in other positions.

Open Up
The woman lies on her back with her ankles around her neck. The man penetrates from above, supporting his weight on his arms or, if he's strong enough, using one hand to support his own weight and the other to hold his lover's legs in place for an added submissive kick. Again, this position can be reversed for strap-on sex.

Reverse Cowgirl
The man lies on his back. The woman then straddles him, facing his feet. The further forward she leans, the more the penis will press into her G-spot. This position can be used for strap-on sex and may stimulate the prostate particularly effectively. However, if you're new to anal, standard cowgirl will probably be easier.

INSPIRATION FOR SEX OUTSIDE THE BEDROOM

- *The kitchen table:* Bend over, and away you go. Just make sure you clean up any crumbs first.

- *The washing machine:* Just hit spin cycle for added vibrations.

- *The sofa:* Kneel on it, lie on it, bend over it—the sofa is probably the most sex versatile piece of furniture, so use it to its full potential. Don't forget that you can use the cushions to help you vary the angle of entry, too.

- *The stairs:* Stand on different stairs from each other and work out which gives you the best angle for ultimate pleasure. Make sure you hold on tight.

- *The desk:* Great for office sex role play, just push the papers to one side and get stuck into each other.

- *Floor cushions:* Imagine you're in a harem or simply use the cushions to change the angles with which you approach each other. You can also buy specially designed sex furniture that looks innocent but offers hidden secrets.

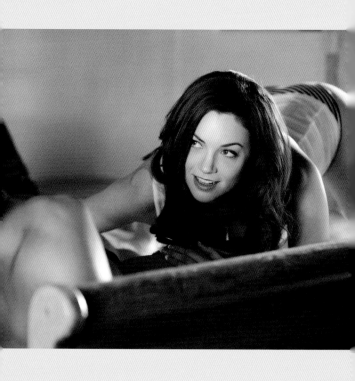

1 · The Morning Horn

STIMULATING MULTIPLE EROGENOUS ZONES at once can be one of the easiest way to ramp up your sex life and speed your lover's climax. If you're lucky enough to wake up and encounter your man's morning horn pressing against you, there's an obvious thing to do: get blowing while he's still asleep. But as with musical instruments that you blow, what you do with your hands is just as important as what you do with your mouth.

Grip your man's shaft with one hand while your lips play up and down the penis from root to tip. Play your fingers up and down the shaft while your thumb rubs up and down the underside of the penis. Let your tongue swirl around the head of the penis, and alternate this with slow, deep sucks: you don't make sweet music by playing a single note, after all.

Use your other hand to stroke your man's inner thighs, cup and stroke his balls, or play with his nipples: if you're not sure which are his favorite erogenous zones (other than the obvious) then ask him—though not while your mouth's full, it's rude. Pay attention to the way that his penis swells as you stroke your lover's erogenous zones: the harder it gets, the more attention you should pay. Speed your movements as he nears climax, and you're likely to help him start the day with a smile.

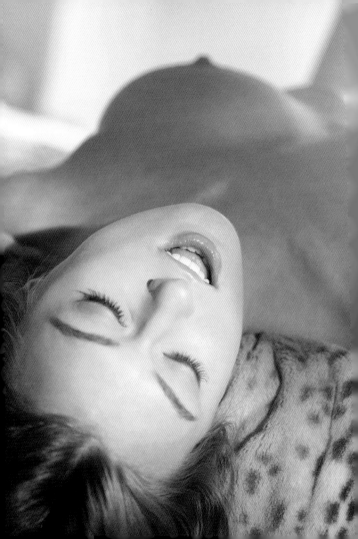

2 · Happy Birthday

ORAL SEX IS BY FAR THE EASIEST WAY for most women to reach climax, and what better a way to deliver a birthday bonus than with a good tongue lashing as soon as she wakes up? Slow, steady movements will often speed climax far more than hard and fast tongue lashes.

Circle your tongue around your lover's clitoris, being careful to avoid the sensitive tip until she's fully warmed up. For many women, hard and fast pressure is far more likely to kill the mood than a softly, softly approach.

Base your movements on her birthday: if she's twenty-one, circle twenty-one times to the left then twenty-one times to the right, and if she's fifty, opt for fifty strokes in each direction. The different approaches will stimulate different areas. Give some love to the clitoral shaft—a miniature version of the shaft of the penis— licking from side to side until she starts to push her clit into your mouth.

Women often prefer constant movements to ever-changing techniques, so once you're moving your tongue in a way that's making her moan, don't change what you're doing unless her boil turns into a simmer. Let her guide your movements with her hands, she knows where she most wants to be stimulated better than anyone, after all.

And don't forget to use your hands as well as your mouth. If she's into G-spot stimulation, crook your finger once you've slid it inside her, and move it back and forth until you find an area that starts to swell. Keep your finger moving over this area as you lick, suck, and breathe over your lover's bits. The more it swells, the more aroused she's getting, but be warned, some women ejaculate through G-spot stimulation, so don't be surprised if you end up with a wet face before you've got anywhere near the shower.

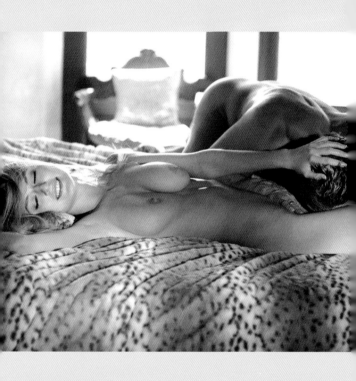

3 · Wake Her Up with Lovers' T

FIRST THING IN THE MORNING is no time for acrobatic antics. Instead, opt for lazy but original positions to help you stimulate your lover in ways that you never have before. The Lovers' T is a great oral sex position that allows the woman to lie back and enjoy herself while her partner kneels comfortably beside her. .

To assume the position, the woman lies on her back and her partner kneels to her side at groin level, leaning forward to plant his face in her most intimate folds. However, rather than trying to get his tongue inside her, the man should focus all his attention on the clitoral shaft. Avoid the sensitive clitoral tip until the woman is super-aroused.

As the woman becomes wet, her partner should slide one or more fingers inside her, and feel around for an area on the upper wall of the vagina that swells when pressed, aka the G-spot. Dual stimulation of the clitoral shaft and G-spot can be incredibly intense for some women.

If she starts arching toward your face, try delicately stimulating the clitoral tip. Use the side of your tongue rather than the tip of your tongue to start with, as this can offer more delicate stimulation. Increase pressure according to the way your lover moves her body.

Of course, if time is really short or the woman simply wants to get more involved, she can increase her pleasure by caressing her breasts and/or nipples, stroking other erogenous zones, adding her hand to her lover's and helping him masturbate her, or bringing a toy into play.

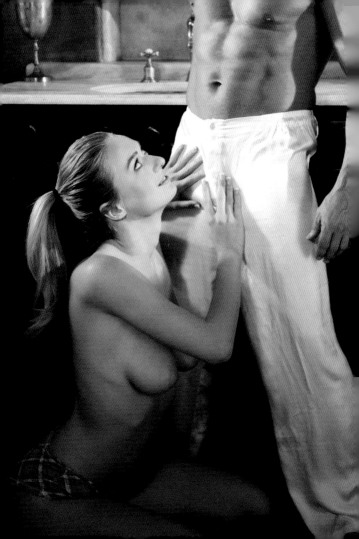

4 · Wake Him Up with Teabagging

STIMULATING MULTIPLE EROGENOUS ZONES at once can be one of the easiest way to ramp up your sex life and speed your lover's climax. If you're lucky enough to wake up and encounter your man's morning horn pressing against you, there's an obvious thing to do: get blowing while he's still asleep. But as with musical instruments that you blow, what you do with your hands is just as important as what you do with your mouth.

Grip your man's shaft with one hand while your lips play up and down the penis from root to tip. Play your fingers up and down the shaft while your thumb rubs up and down the underside of the penis. Let your tongue swirl around the head of the penis, and alternate this with slow, deep sucks: you don't make sweet music by playing a single note, after all.

Use your other hand to stroke your man's inner thighs, cup and stroke his balls, or play with his nipples: if you're not sure which are his favorite erogenous zones (other than the obvious) then ask him—though not while your mouth's full, it's rude. Pay attention to the way that his penis swells as you stroke your lover's erogenous zones: the harder it gets, the more attention you should pay. Speed your movements as he nears climax, and you're likely to help him start the day with a smile.

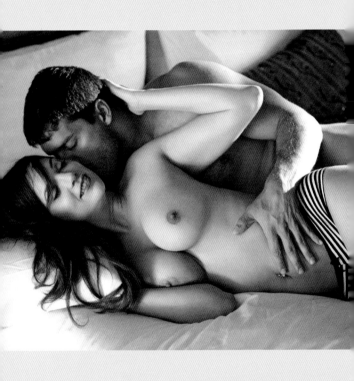

5 · Alarm Call

THANKS TO THE WONDERS of shrinking technology and genius engineers, it's now possible to get sex toys of all shapes and sizes serving a multitude of functions, including an alarm clock. At the time this deck was published, there were two alarm clock vibrators on the market for women (and one in development for men, but you'll have to wait a while yet—sorry guys). These slip inside a woman's pajama bottoms or panties, pressed against her most intimate areas, and rouse her from her sleep with an ever-more-insistent buzz.

If you're short on time, what's better than an alarm clock that starts foreplay off for you?

Once she starts to wake, cuddle into your lover from behind, cupping her breasts, caressing her buttocks, and kissing the side of her neck.

As she starts to respond to your touch, move your hands ever nearer her alarm clock, softly tracing her inner thighs with your fingertips and slowly circling the pubic mound until her hips are raised off the bed and you can slide a finger inside her, apply more pressure to the toy, or both, depending on her preferences.

The alarm clock vibrator is a clitoral toy, worn externally. This means that snuggling up to her from behind gives easy access to slide inside her: her muscular spasms at the toy's ministrations teamed with her buttocks wriggling back against you should ensure you both have a passionate start to the day.

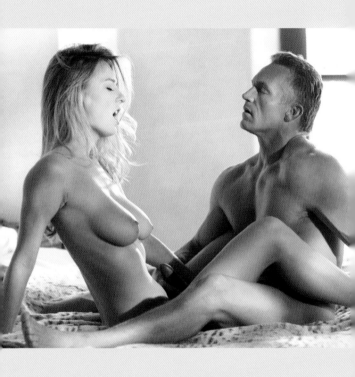

6 · Making Juice

RENOWNED SEXPERT LOU PAGET first came up with the fantastic name "Squeezing the Orange" to describe a manual sex technique that can help speed a man's climax. First, lubricate the penis thoroughly. Then use one hand on your lover's shaft, stroking up and down, and cup your other hand. Move your cupped hand to the head of your lover's penis and grasp the well-lubricated head in your palm, swirling it from side to side as your other hand continues to pulse up and down your lover's shaft.

But this isn't just about giving your lover some breakfast juice. He will be using a machine to make juice too, namely, your favorite vibrator, but with a twist. Rather than using the sex toy to thrust in and out of you, your lover just needs to press the vibrate button and hold it still: something that he'll probably be relieved about as he's likely to be rather distracted by your ministrations. He needs to make sure that he holds the sex toy in such a way that it's easy for you to grind against it (using lube will make this more comfortable unless you're already wet). By grinding against the toy, you're not only in control of when and how much stimulation you get, but you'll also increase blood flow to the pelvic region, which can boost orgasmic chances.

You may find that sitting opposite each other with your legs spread and crossed over each other's offers the easiest access for mutual play. Alternatively, you may want to kneel to your lover's side with him lying flat on his back. Pick a position that's comfortable for you both, then enjoy pleasuring each other. There's no need to feel self-conscious about grinding against the toy. Chances are, it'll be a serious turn-on for your partner, assuming you're both comfortable with toys. If anything, it'll make sure you get your morning juice fast.

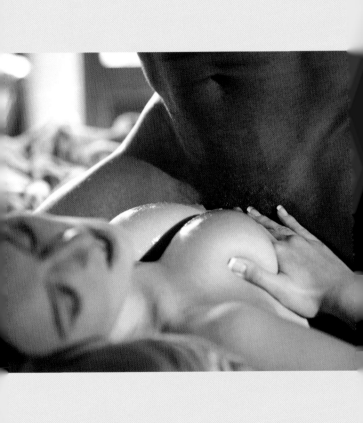

7 · A Pair Of Fried Eggs

IF YOU'RE NOT IN the mood for a sausage breakfast but want to give your lover a treat, how about a pair of fried eggs instead (an analogy that's stuck with me after being affectionately applied to my own rather diminutive breasts)? Yes, we're talking breasts here, which are generally the object of receiving rather than giving pleasure during sex. Here, they take a more active role teamed with lube.

Drizzle lube between your breasts, making sure to cover your cleavage liberally. Now, get your partner to straddle your body, add more lube to his penis (a process that will also help ensure he's hard enough to enjoy himself fully) and ask him to slide between your boobs and start thrusting. You'll need to hold your boobs together to create enough friction (and yes, even if you've got small boobs it can be fun–you'll just need to squeeze them together more tightly and possibly use your hand to close the gap.)

Add more lube as required and, if your man's into it, add some dirty talk to the equation to speed things along. If you want to indulge in oral too, simply bend your head forward to receive the head of the penis when he thrusts toward you. Otherwise, encourage him to give you a 'pearl necklace' (ejaculate on your breasts) or, if you're short on time and can't shower afterward, simply finish him off with your hands.

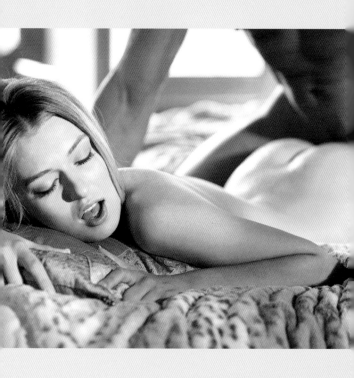

8 · Breakfast Buns

APPLY LUBE to the crease of the buttocks rather than the anus—when your man thrusts, he needs to be aiming upwards (towards your back, with the culmination of the thrust being at the coccyx at the base of the spine) rather than downwards (towards your anus/vagina). Slip a condom onto your lover so that you're safe even if he does accidentally get his aim wrong (all too easy to happen when you're dealing with lubed-up bits).

Liberally cover your man's member in lube then lie in the spooning position with your lover behind you, and position his penis between your buttocks. Now, he simply needs to start thrusting to get his kicks. Clenching your buttocks as he thrusts will add extra sensation.

While he thrusts, your lover can cup your breasts or move his hand lower down to stroke your clitoris and cup your mons, so that you can both enjoy your breakfast buns together. Alternatively, you can use your fingers on yourself, hold a vibrator against your clitoris, or use a Rabbit style vibrator for dual clitoral and G-spot stimulation. Try timing it with your lover's thrusts if you want a more connected experience.

As he nears climax, he can either pull away or ejaculate over your back and buttocks. However, do be extremely careful if opting for the latter: sexual fluids have a habit of spreading and you need to ensure you keep yourself safe.

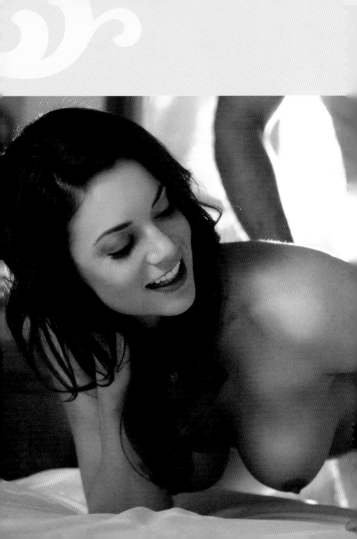

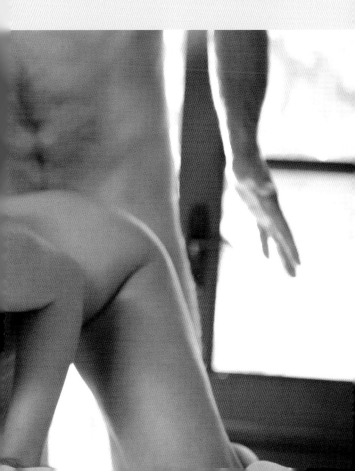

9 · Pain au Chocolat

SEEKING A BREAKFAST that's a bit more kinky? How about combining spanking with anal play for a truly naughty wake-up call? Being spanked releases endorphins, the body's natural pain killers that can lead to an ecstatic high if properly managed. Start by spanking lightly and gradually increase the pressure to help the endorphins flow with ease. Once your lover is wriggling in anticipation, throw the anal play into the mix for a double-whammy of kinky fun.

The anus is densely packed with nerve endings that, if stimulated in the right way, can lead to intense pleasure. Although some people enjoy anal penetration, it can take time for the anus to relax suffi- ciently for it to be comfortable. Focusing your attention on the 'rosebud' instead can bring great pleasure without the same risk of pain (of course, if you're into more hard-core submissive/domination play, pain may be arousing, but do make sure you keep yourself and your partner safe by using lots of lubricant and going carefully to avoid ripping or tearing the anal tissue.)

There are numerous ways to stimulate the anus. You can lightly circle your finger around it, rub two or more fingers over the entire anal region (pressing into a man's perineum can be thrilling for some as it stimulates the prostate [aka the male G-spot] from the outside) or use a dental dam and rim (lick) your partner. This should not be done without a dam, as otherwise you can expose yourself to hepatitis, e-coli, and numerous other infections, not all of which are STIs.

Alternate spanking with anal worship for a delicious pain/pleasure hybrid (assuming that's your thing, of course).

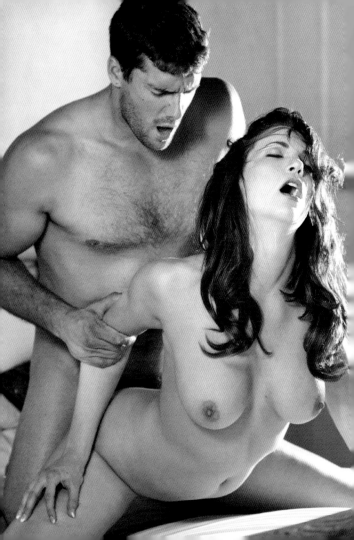

10 · Morning Breathless

ALTHOUGH IT'S NICE TO BELIEVE that love conquers all, first thing in the morning is never the time that your breath smells its sweetest. However, morning breath doesn't have to hamper your passion. Instead, avoid the problem with some hot doggy style sex, with the woman on all fours and the man kneeling behind her. This position is great for quickies, as it allows easy access for the woman to masturbate during sex, and it's just as simple for the man to hold a vibrator against her clit.

Add an extra frisson by positioning yourselves in front of a mirror: the additional visual stimulation should help both of you feel frisky. Where you position the mirror is entirely up to you. You might want to face it, so you can maintain eye contact with your lover despite your distance. You may choose a side-on position so that you can see the sex act in full. If you've got multiple mirrors, you can even position them to reflect the business end as well as your faces.

If the woman lowers her upper body to the bed or floor, keeping her buttocks in the air, it will deepen penetration, which can be a good way to speed the man's climax, as well as the woman's if she enjoys G-spot stimulation. If doggy style offers sex that is too deep, the woman simply needs to lie flat rather than being on all fours. Or opt for an interim position with the woman lying flat but with a pillow under her pelvis. Whichever method you choose, if the woman flexes her Kegel muscles, it will add extra stimulation for you both and enhance your chances of a speedy orgasm. Then brush your teeth and have a kiss and a cuddle. Intimacy is an important part of sex too, and will help you start your day feeling loved up and happy.

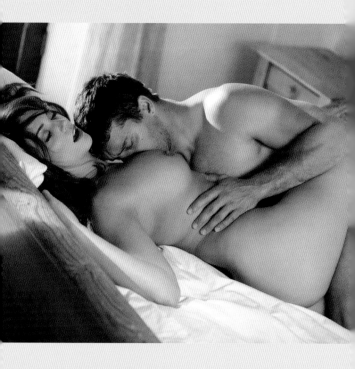

11 · Cutting It Close

IF YOU'RE AFTER FAST SEX with mutual pleasure, clitoral stimulation is a necessity. Sadly, it's not always easy to stimulate the whole of the clitoris, through sex, which can mean it takes longer for a woman to reach climax than a man. However, scissoring during sex is a great way to level up the amount of pleasure you're both getting, as it allows constant clitoral stimulation throughout sex and means that the woman can position herself to best hit the erotic hotspots she wants to.

Start by lying on your side, facing each other. The man then penetrates the woman, who then slides one of her legs in between his legs so that they are scissored together.

Thrusting is less vigorous than in other positions, but the woman can rock her hips and grind back against the man to deepen penetration. Arching her back and matching her partner's thrusts will also help angle her pelvis in such a way as to deepen penetration. She can also flex her Kegel muscles to increase friction and make sex more pleasurable for both of you. You can cover the woman's breasts or man's chest in lube to make the entire experience more slippery and wild. Both partners can squeeze each other's buttocks or indulge in light anal play during sex, or for a more sensual and romantic twist, you can rub and massage each other's shoulders or backs as you have sex: talk about a relaxing start to the day.

This position allows lots of scope for intimate sex, with kissing and caressing throughout. This makes it a great loving way to start the day that should help you both get your oats and keep you feeling satisfied until lunchtime and beyond.

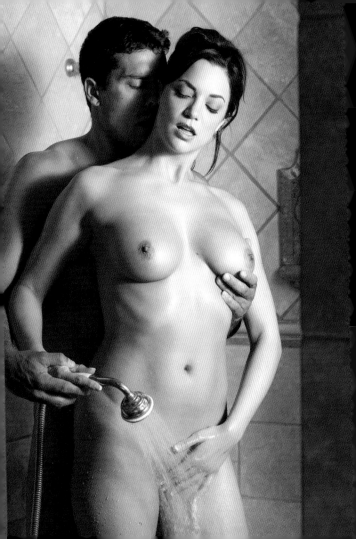

12 · Showered with Affection

TAKING YOUR LOVEMAKING OUTSIDE THE BEDROOM can inject fresh passion into your relationship, and if you're short on time first thing, what better way of multi-tasking than teaming your morning shower with some first-thing frolicking?

Not only is the shower perfect for sex standing up, giving plenty of surfaces to lean against, but you can also use the shower head to spray over each other's erogenous zones, which can be particularly effective on the clitoris. However, don't spray water up the vagina as it can (ironically) make the woman dry up.

Start by giving each other a thorough soaping. Use a wet wash cloth: the texture may provide you with an extra thrill. Massage soap into every other inch of your lover's skin until they're bubbling with anticipation.

You have various options position-wise. Both of you can stand facing the same direction with the woman in front of the man. The man then slides in from behind and uses one hand to focus the shower head over the woman's clit and the other to caress her breasts and torso.

Alternatively, the woman can stand leaning forward from the waist, with her arms braced against the wall, and the man can penetrate, again from behind. This will make penetration deeper and allows the woman to push back harder against her partner, which is great if she's into G-spot stimulation or you like hard, fast sex.

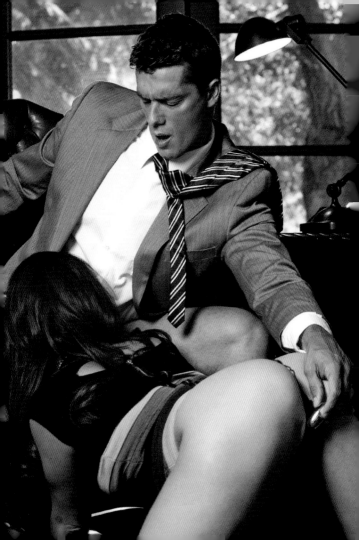

13 · Diet Cock Break

THERE'S SOMETHING INNATELY NAUGHTY about having sex during the day. Imagining everyone else at work while you're sneaking out to have a quickie can really make your pulse race, and if you add a hint of danger, it can be even more intoxicating.

If you're inclined toward an exhibitionist streak, take a break from work together for some outdoor fun. When you pack your bag for work, make sure one of you includes a bullet vibrator. Pick a model that's quiet because you're going to be taking it out and about and don't want a noisy buzz to draw attention to your naughtiness. There are numerous small vibrators disguised as everyday objects, from a lipstick to a pen, which will spare any blushes if it falls out of your bag. It's also worth the woman packing a spare pair of tights or stockings: you may end up laddering yours and don't want your outfit to give away your erotic adventure.

When it gets to the agreed time, make your way to the Diet Cock Break location. It could be a discreet alleyway, some nearby woods, or even be a deserted office in one of your workplaces, but only if you're extremely sure you won't get caught and/or there's a lock on the door: it's not worth losing your job over some quickie fun.

Wherever you choose, once you arrive, there's one objective: oral sex for him and toy fun for her with the added exhibitionist thrill for both of you. The woman should get on her knees and start sucking, having first slipped the vibe into her undies. Oral sex can be as hot to give as to receive, particularly if you focus on showing your lover exactly how much he means to you with your lips and tongue, and of course, the vibrator on the woman's clit is sure to add an extra buzz.

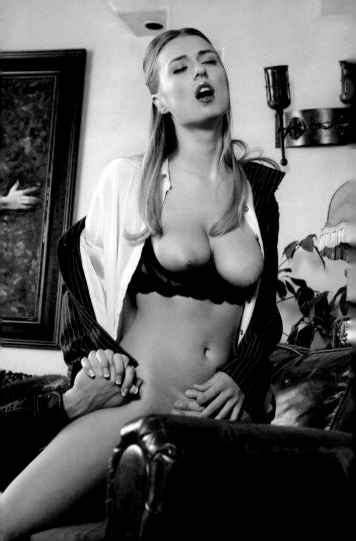

14 · Box Lunch

IF YOU'VE TAKEN A Diet Cock Break (#13), it's only fair to have a Box Lunch, too. Yes, we're talking a lunchtime oral session for her. The easiest way to hit all of a woman's hot spots is to allow her to set the pace. Woman-on-top oral is ideal for this, as it not only allows her to grind her clitoris into the man's face, but also makes it easy for her to pull away if the sensation is too much. The man can also introduce his fingers to the equation.

The man should try different oral techniques until he finds one that hits the spot. Once he has, continue with the same technique unless she requests otherwise. The man can try the following:

- Running his tongue over the clitoral shaft
- Lapping up the left hand side of the labia and down the right hand side, and vice versa
- Circling the tongue around the clit
- Softly sucking the clit
- Penetrating the vagina with his tongue
- Using the underside or side of his tongue to lick the clitoral tip (It's far gentler so this move is ideal if the woman has a particularly sensitive clit.)

Commit the techniques that work to memory and with any luck, it'll speed her orgasm during oral, whether you're short for time or not.

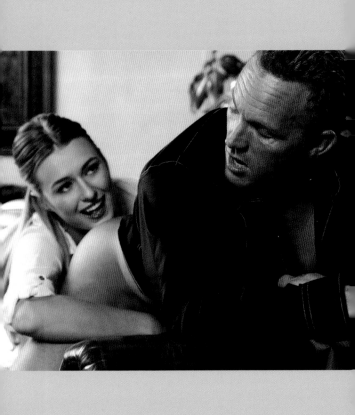

15 · Toss His Salad

SOMETIMES YOU WANT SOMETHING DIFFERENT for lunch, which is where tossing his salad (aka rimming) enters the arena. While it's not to everyone's preference, many people find oral stimulation of the anus to be deeply thrilling. However, you should ensure that you use a dental dam (a square of latex used to cover the area), as otherwise you can expose yourself not just to sexually transmitted infections but also e-coli and other bacteria.

Draw a non-reversible letter, such as L or R, on the dental dam with non-toxic indelible ink. That way, if it pings out of your hand during use (which is all too easy to happen) you'll know which side was the 'safe' side and can continue to use it without any fears that it's facing the wrong way. And it should go without saying that the man should ensure he's thoroughly cleaned first: you don't want any noxious odors putting your partner off her lunch.

There are various positions to choose from. The man can kneel on all fours with his partner behind him for easy access. She can then use one hand to stretch the dam over his anus while the other hand gets to work masturbating her lover's shaft. Alternatively, the man can stand, bracing his hands against a wall, with his partner kneeling behind him. Or the man can lie on his back with his ankles over his head. No matter which position you choose, the woman will find it much easier to do if the man holds his buttocks apart with his hands.

Once in position, the woman simply holds the dam in place and starts licking and penetrating the man's anus with her tongue, using a lubed-up hand to stroke his shaft as she does so. The combined sensations of anal exploring and masturbation of the shaft should help take him over the edge in record time.

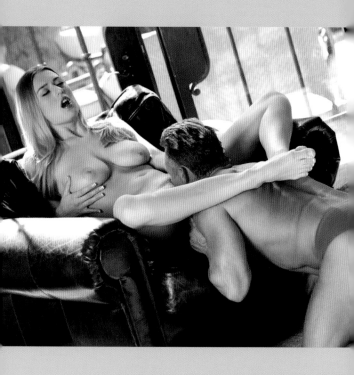

16 · Stuffed Sandwich

WHEN YOU WANT a lunchtime treat that's really filling, try the Stuffed Sandwich. All you need to do is take a toy of your choice and combine it with cunnilingus. Some popular options include the following:

- *Crystal dildos:* Made from specially treated glass that's designed to be all-but-unbreakable, these can be chilled in the fridge or warmed in a cup of water to add an extra twist.

- *Perspex dildos:* A cheaper alternative to crystal dildos, these can be used in similar ways, though they hold heat and cold less effectively than crystal.

- *Silicone dildos:* Silicone is a hugely popular material in modern sex toys as it's free of phthalates. It warms with your body and is available in almost any shape you can imagine.

- *Metal dildos:* These are heavier than most dildos. The weight can add extra oomph to G-spot stimulation.

- *Wooden dildos:* Made using techniques that ensure there's no risk of splinters, these are eco-friendly and naturally antibacterial. They retain warmth, so they are great if you don't like cold toys.

The man should use lubricant to insert the dildo, checking that he likes the taste before applying it, then let his tongue get to work. The woman can guide his movements with her hand to speed her progress toward climax.

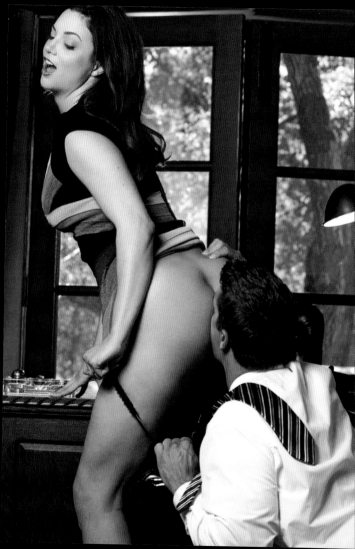

17 · Ass-Kissing Lunch

IF THE MAN GETS his salad tossed, it's only fair that the woman gets an Ass-kissing Lunch, too. As with rimming a man, using a dental dam is essential. Stroking the man's shaft should be replaced with thumbing the woman's well lubricated clitoris and sliding one or more fingers inside her.

Position-wise, you have various options. The woman can kneel on all fours, doggie style, parting her buttocks with her hands to allow easy access. The man then kneels behind her, stretching the dental dam over anus, her then diving in, using his fingers to thrust in and out of her vagina or press against her G-spot.

Alternatively, the woman can lie face down on the bed or floor, making access easier by spreading her cheeks. The man can lie on top of her or kneel to the side, depending on which allows him to explore more freely (which can vary depending on where the woman is lying).

If she wants more control, the woman can stand over the man, leaning against a wall and bracing herself against it while he sits between her legs and works his magic. Or if both partners are into female domination, try face sitting, in which the woman literally sits on the man's face with her anus over his mouth. This can stifle the man's breathing so handle with care, though some men do like the sensation of being stifled, and as long as he can breathe enough to be safe, it's not necessarily a bad thing.

Depending on the position you choose, you might want to incorporate a toy into proceedings to add extra stimulation. If time is of the essence, it's worth hitting as many erogenous zones as possible. The tri-gasmic bliss of combined anal, vaginal, and clitoral stimulation should help her come far more rapidly than stimulating one erogenous zone in isolation.

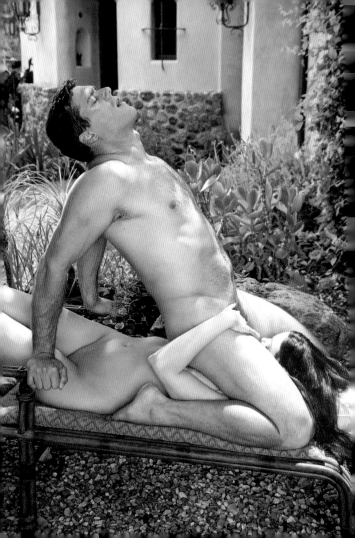

18 · 12 O'Cock

FOR FAST AND FURIOUS FELLATIO, you can't get much better than 12 O'Cock because it puts the man completely in control. Better yet, once the woman has mastered her gag reflex, all she has to do is keep her mouth open and let the man do all the work.

This can work in various positions. If the man can come when he's standing (some men find it tricky) the woman can simply kneel in front of him. If not, the woman can lie on the bed or floor and the man can get onto all fours over her face, using pillows to raise her face to the appropriate level. A sofa offers scope for fun too: the woman sits on the sofa while the man kneels on the sofa with his penis, pretty obviously, at mouth level.

Once in position, the woman should open her mouth and guard her teeth with her lips to ensure she doesn't inadvertently graze the man's intimate parts. The man then slides inside and thrusts away to his heart's content. However, he should be careful not to thrust too deeply, particularly to start with, as she may end up gagging.

The woman can deal with her gag reflex in various ways. She can practice with a courgette or dildo so that her throat gets used to the sensation (or indeed, use her partner for practice. He's unlikely to complain. Flaring the nostrils raises the soft palate at the back of the throat, which can minimise the risk of gagging. If a woman has a hard time controlling her gag reflex, she can simply use her hand to steer the penis into the side of her cheek instead of down her throat.

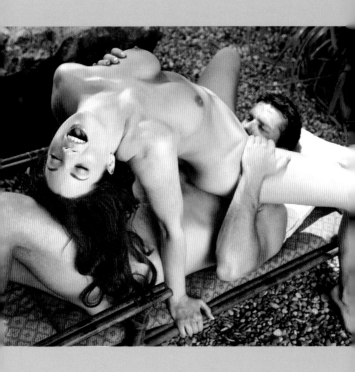

19 · Eating In

ALTHOUGH EATING OUT ALLOWS lots of scope for naughtiness, eating In gives you a lot more freedom of movement, so take advantage by indulging in some mutual oral for lunch. Add an extra frisson by taking your oral pleasuring outside the bedroom. If you always have sex in the same place, it's easy to get stuck in a rut, but by changing the location, it's easier to change the sex that you have, too. Variety is often a great way to fire the libido and speed orgasm.

One of you lies back on the sofa with your head on the arm. The other gets on top, sixty-nine style, holding on to thea sofa for support if required. Place a cushion underneath your lover's hips to best angle his or her bits toward your mouth.

Alternatively, try mutual oral on the living room floor. The trick to making this super exciting is passion: grab your partner as soon as he or she comes into the house, peel his or her clothes off, and drag him or her onto the floor in a heated kissing session. Kissing is much underestimated and is often the first thing to fade in a long-term relationship. We release pheromones through our upper lips that identify how biologically compatible we are with a partner (which is why two kisses that are identical in technique can feel very different from different people). If you're biologically attracted to each other, you're missing a trick if you don't exploit those pheromones to the fullest. Kiss for at least five minutes, then use the remaining ten or so to indulge in mutual oral. With any luck, the kissing will have stimulated saliva flow and, as a general rule, the wetter the better applies with oral, so it'll make the oral encounter hotter, too.

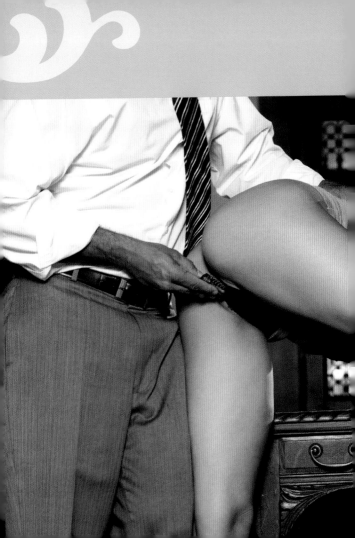

20 · Finger Sandwich

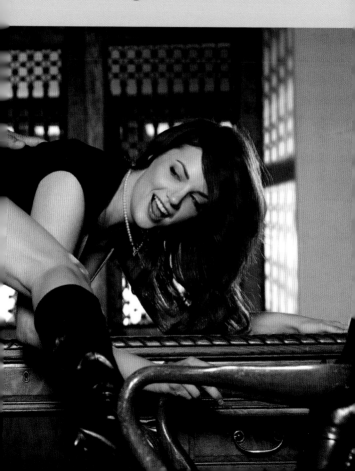

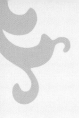

20 · Finger Sandwich

SOMETIMES YOU WANT a light lunch, and this is where the Finger Sandwich comes in: an easy way to enjoy a quick midday thrill, and all you need is a vibrating finger ring. A finger ring is like a cock ring but, as the name suggests, it's smaller so it can fit on your finger. They come with varying types of vibrators but generally tend to offer fairly mild vibrations, so they're great if you're new to toys.

The location is up to you. One of the joys of fingering is that, unlike sex, it can be done extremely discreetly, if you dress appropriately. The woman should wear a skirt with stockings but no underwear to make access as easy as possible. That way, you can choose to meet each other in a local park, discreet alley, or even a busy bar. Finger rings tend to be very quiet, so unless you're somewhere extremely quiet, such as a library or museum, you won't be overheard (assuming the woman can keep her moans under control). Alternatively, you can meet at home and, depending on your preference, opt for a wild fingering in the hall as soon as your lover gets home.

Don't go straight for the clitoral tip unless you're certain your lover wants you to, as this can be too intense for some women. Instead, let the vibrations stimulate the entire pubic area and vulva, sliding one or more fingers inside your lover as she gets more aroused to sandwich her clit between the finger ring and your fingers inside her. The double stimulation will help speed her orgasm: a fast, light lunchtime treat.

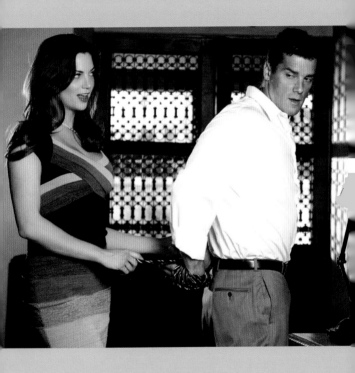

21 · Tied-Up Afternoon

LOOKING FOR SOMETHING TO add a kinky frisson to your lunch hour? Bondage against the clock could be just what you're looking for. This isn't the time to get into Japanese rope bondage or elaborate scenes involving complex power exchange role plays. Instead, opt for a good old fashioned pair of handcuffs teamed with your favorite sex acts.

You could opt for mutual pleasure, restraining your partner before having sex in a position you know gets him or her off while he or she struggles against the bonds. You could choose to take your lover to the brink with some exquisite oral, telling him or her not to come until you say so: denying orgasm can often provide a thrill as your lover struggles to obey his or her orders. Or you could opt for something more animal, with your lover in a more obviously submissive role. The way you play it is entirely up to the pair of you, but do make sure it is all mutually consensual.

It's a good idea to choose to use a safe word: a word other than "no" or "stop" that indicates you must stop what you're doing immediately. Many people use the traffic light system, with red meaning "stop," yellow meaning "slow down" and green meaning "go ahead."

Set an alarm for your activities. Knowing you've got a time limit to stick to can add an extra sexy tension to proceedings.

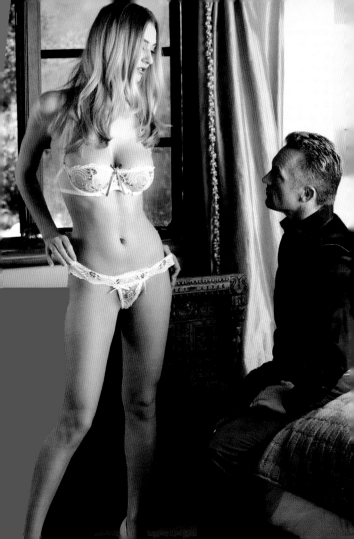

22 · Afternoon Delight

IF YOU'VE GOT A FULL LUNCH HOUR to play with, go for the classic if not clichéd Afternoon Delight by finding a cheap motel and renting a room for an hour. (If you can't find anywhere that rents by the hour, opt for the cheapest motel you can find. You can always come back later.) Pick somewhere you wouldn't usually go to, where you're unlikely to bump into anyone you know, to allow yourself the aphrodisiac of anonymity. This is going to be one hell of an hour!

Think about the things that you've always wanted to do, and get your partner to do the same. It might be a sex act or trying out a new toy. You might even choose to indulge in a role-play, such as horny business-woman and eager-to-please room service attendant or escort and client. If you opt for the fantasy approach, stay in character from the moment you meet your lover at the hotel to the moment that you leave.

It doesn't matter what you choose to do. Half of the fun to be had is in the chat you have with your lover about how you're going to spend your time, before you get to the hotel. (Ideally, plan it a while in advance to give you both time to let the ideas simmer and stock up on any props that you require.)

Once you're in your hotel room, let yourselves go wild. No one you know can hear you. There is no one around to judge you. Hell, you can even use a fake name such as Mr. and Mrs. Smith if you need that level of anonymity to abandon yourself. Relax, go with the flow, and you'll truly make the most of the limited time that you have together.

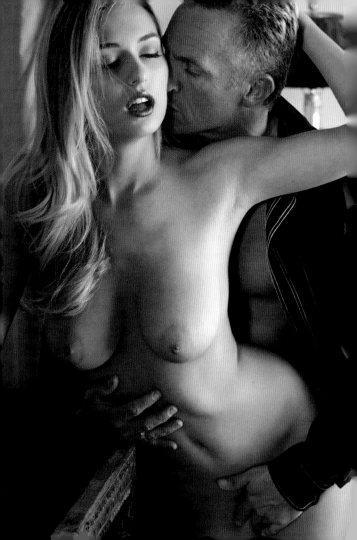

23 · Sneaky Sandwich

SHORT ON TIME but simply have to have each other? Opt for a Sneaky Sandwich so that you can both enjoy a satisfying lunch. Where you opt to eat it is entirely up to you. If you're feeling exhibitionist, it'll work in a discreet alleyway. If that's just a tad too wild for you, a bathroom stall at a restaurant offers an alternative. And if you're able to meet at home, you could simply do it against the wall as soon as you see each other.

To get into the Sneaky Sandwich, the woman stands in front of a wall, bracing her arms against it and sticking her bum out. This not only gives her lover a great view, but also positions her so that penetration will be as deep as possible and her G-spot will be hit with every stroke. (If a woman doesn't enjoy G-spot stimulation, she simply needs to stand slightly straighter to make the angle more comfortable).

The man then stands behind her and slides in, using lubricant if required, with his hand on her pubic mound and the pads of his fingers on her clitoris. He can stretch his thumb out to stimulate her internal clitoris too, pressing into the belly gently until he finds an area that makes her wriggle back in delight (do make sure it's delight, not discomfort though: ask if you're remotely unsure).

The woman can add extra pleasure to the experience by clenching her Kegel muscles as the man thrusts. Flexing the Kegels will also increase blood flow to the area, thus intensifying her orgasm too. The man should maintain constant contact with the pubic mound and clitoris, following his lover's verbal and non-verbal cues as to pressure and positioning. By having the clitoris, mons, and G-spot sandwiched between hand and penis, the woman should find it much easier to come.

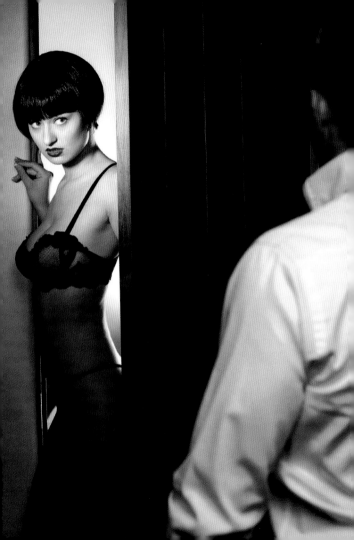

24 · Lunchtime Liaison

AS TIME GOES ON, it can be easy to take your lover for granted, but the Lunchtime Liaison offers a quick and easy way to make things fresh again because you'll be meeting as strangers. You will need a little planning to enjoy this as you'll both need a flattering outfit and wig that you can change into quickly that makes you look as different as possible. You should be able to find both in thrift shops or drug stores, so this needn't be expensive. Agree to meet somewhere that you wouldn't usually go and a specific time. You don't want to pick up the wrong person by mistake.

When you meet, you can take the role play in whatever direction you want. One of you could ask the other for directions, only to be met with a flirtatious response. One of you could be an escort, a spy, or even a time traveller from the future: whatever works for you both. You could have a complex sexy conversation before grabbing a quick, heated moment together before you part, or you could simply meet and start kissing without saying a single word. Pick something that turns both of you on–feeling self-conscious isn't sexy–and let the encounter play out naturally.

The trick here is to see your partner with fresh eyes, so don't make reference to your everyday life together or use any jokes you may share. Instead, pay attention to the person who's in front of you. Look at him or her as if you've never seen him or her before, and remind yourself why you fell for this person in the first place. Then find somewhere private to show how much you like what you see.

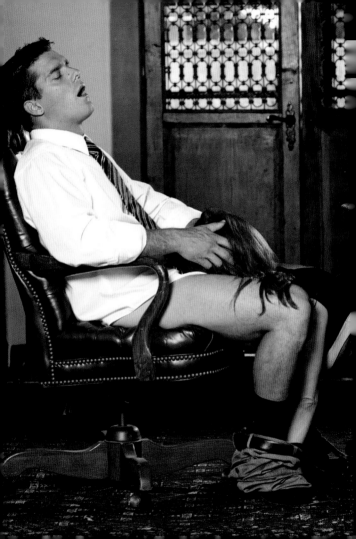

25 · Take Dicktation

AS THE NAME SUGGESTS, this entails getting under your lover's desk and performing fellatio. The space limitations mean that your movements may be hampered, but this just gives you a chance to experiment with different techniques.

While the woman is down there, the man has various options. He can watch his lover's movements if he's not worried about being seen. He can continue working on his computer, which can be arousing for some submissive women who get off on serving their lovers (within sex, at least).

As with all oral, it'll be faster if the woman uses one or both hands as well as her mouth to stimulate her lover. Different techniques to try include the following:

- Licking the penis from root to tip
- Sucking just the tip of the penis into the mouth and bobbing the head back and forth
- Working the shaft having first lubricated it well with saliva while sucking the tip as above
- Circling the tongue around the head of the penis
- Playing with the man's balls while sucking the penis
- Sliding your lips to the base of the penis, flaring the nostrils to retract the tonsils and help avoid the gag reflex kicking in

Try to incorporate at least one new technique to add the element of surprise.

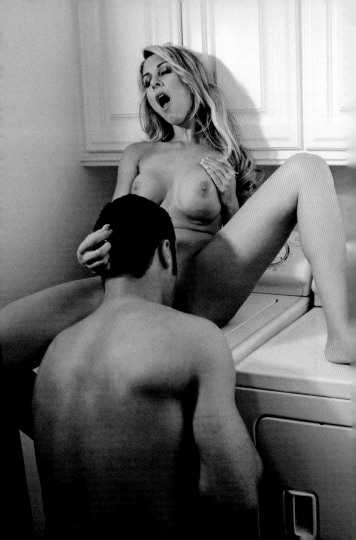

26 · Wash-and-Go

IF YOU'RE LUCKY ENOUGH to have a rapid setting on your washing machine, the Wash-and-Go is a classic way to speed your chances of mutual orgasm. All you need to do is set the spin cycle going, then have sex over the washing machine. (Put a load of laundry in while you're at it—you don't want to waste water.)

When it comes to positions, you have various options. Depending on the size and position of your washing machine, the easiest position is most likely to involve the woman bending over the washing machine while her partner penetrates her from behind. Generally speaking, the vibrations will travel through the front casing of the washing machine, making it easy to ride the wave. (Do make sure you've seen your washing machine on spin cycle before. You don't want to discover that it shakes itself across the floor at the point it smashes into your pudenda!)

Alternatively, if you don't have a counter top in the way, blocking the vibrations of the washing machine, the man can sit on top of the washing machine. The woman then sits on top of him, facing outward, then you both let the washing machine do all the jiggling for you. The man can make it more intense for the woman by putting his hand over her pubic mound and clitoris, so she can feel the vibrations everywhere it matters.

As a third option, the man can sit on top of the washing machine and the woman can straddle him, squatting on top of the man and using her thigh muscles to raise and lower herself on top of him. By leaning forward to press her clit against his belly, she'll be able to enjoy the vibrations as they ripple through her man's body.

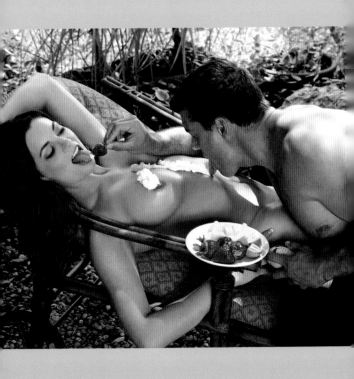

27 · Naked Lunch

MULTI-TASKING IS ALWAYS A good way to save some time, and never more so than with the Naked Lunch. As the name suggests, it simply involves stripping off, then eating lunch off each other's bodies. Get more creative than the traditional squirt of whipped cream or drizzled honey by choosing from one of the following:

- *Fresh fruit platter:* Cover yourself in strawberries, pineapple, and kiwi fruit. This naked lunch could lead to more oral pleasures in the future.

- *Sushi:* Eating sushi off a naked body is known as Nyotaimori if the platter is female and Nantaimori if male. This is quickie food play, so simply make sure you're clean wherever you apply the sushi. You can pour soy sauce into your navel for dipping should you so wish. Careful where you put the wasabi.

- *Afternoon tease:* For a kitsch treat, opt for miniature afternoon tea—think scones and jam, tiny sandwiches, and mini chocolate eclairs. Just make sure you're careful to lick up every single one of those crumbs.

- *Ice cream sundae:* For a sweet-toothed lover, an ice cream sundae can be a real treat if you can cope with the chilling thrill. Add sauce and a cherry as you so wish.

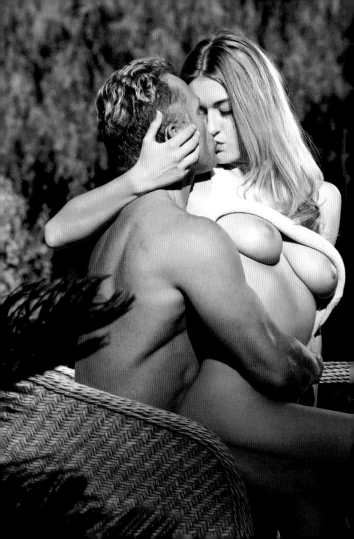

28 · Lazy Lunch

IF THE MAN'S HAD a hard morning at work, and the woman is feeling more active, this position lets him sit back and enjoy himself while she does all the work–but both of you should get your kicks regardless.

The man sits in the middle of the sofa, to allow lots of scope for easy position changes. The woman then sits on his lap, facing away from him, using her legs to control her thrusts up and down. At the same time, she uses one (or more) hands to masturbate. (If the woman has long nails, this can prove dangerous should you move to rapid thrusts, so handle with care).

You can simply continue in this position until you both reach climax– possibly adding an adult movie to the equation if porn films turn you both on. However, should you wish to dial-up some changes, there are various options for speedy sex that the sofa makes so much easier. The woman can turn around to face the man, straddling him on the sofa and leaning forward to grind her clit against his pubic mound or belly.

If you want harder or deeper penetration, the woman can move to lie over the end of the sofa and the man can approach from behind for doggie-style sex with the added bonus of giving the woman something to hold on to so she can drive back further. If you opt for this position, the woman can masturbate or use a toy to ensure she gets the clitoral stimulation she needs.

And if you want the ultimate lazy option for the man, he can lie flat on his back with his lover on top. Rather than staying upright, the woman moves to lie flat on top of the man and gently grinds and rocks her way to orgasmic bliss, finishing off by riding her lover hard until he reaches climax.

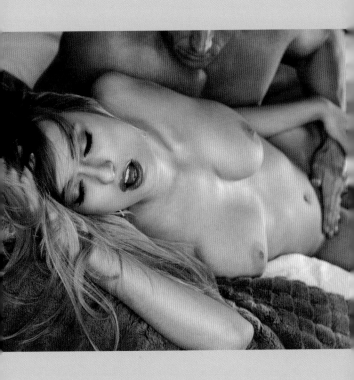

29 · Filling Lunch

IF YOU'VE ENJOYED A Stuffed Sandwich (see #16), a Filling Lunch may also appeal. However, this time, instead of teaming oral with dildo use, you're teaming penetrative sex with vibrator use. Unlike the tongue, the penis won't go numb too quickly from vibrations unless you're using a toy that seriously packs a punch.

Not for the faint hearted, a Filling Lunch is best if the woman enjoys the sensation of being stretched and ideally, gets off on G-spot stimulation, too. Indeed, it's best avoided by women who don't enjoy G-spot stimulation, as it's almost impossible to miss it with this technique.

Start by having sex, either doggie style or spooning, depending on whether you want a raw, animal session or a more loving, kinky experience. Then, once the man is fully inside the woman, she should introduce the toy of her choice into her vagina, too. Take it slowly and remember to guide it carefully alongside the man's penis. Only take it as far as is comfortable. The woman continues to hold the toy as the man thrusts alongside it (alternatively, use a clean anal toy with a flared base to avoid it getting stuck).

Once you're both comfortable with the sensation, turn the vibrations on and enjoy the ride as you both feel the buzz together.

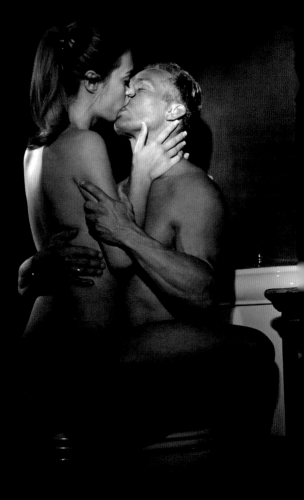

30 · Bathroom Bliss

THERE'S SOMETHING INHERENTLY NAUGHTY about night time. Whether it's because the dark makes us crave security, because we feel more vulnerable, or we simply like the idea of being masked from prying eyes by darkness, there's a reason most dates happen at night. And if the mood strikes when you're out and about, don't think you necessarily have to drag your lover home for an early night. Instead, take advantage of the nearest rest room you can find.

Pick somewhere with multiple stalls–you don't want to keep anyone waiting whose need is greater than yours (this goes doubly for handicap bathrooms). Although they may be enticingly spacious, you don't want to be the person who leaves a disabled person in discomfort because you're banging in the only handicap stall in the vicinity.) Generally speaking, women's bathrooms have a more pleasant aroma than men's. As such, the woman should first "scope out" the area to ensure there are no women in the bathroom who will take offence at a man being in the room (not to mention the noises from inside the stall). Once the coast is clear, the man should get into the stall.

If you want to be as discreet as possible, the man can sit on the toilet with his legs resting against the door and the woman can straddle him, facing forward, so that only her feet appear beneath the door.

For a more shameless encounter, the man can stand, and the woman can drop to her knees to perform fellatio, using her hands for extra stimulation; or the woman can stand and the man can kneel to perform cunnilingus. Alternatively, you could have a mutual manual session leaving both of you sated. Whichever option you choose, there's one more thing to remember: wash your hands when you're done.

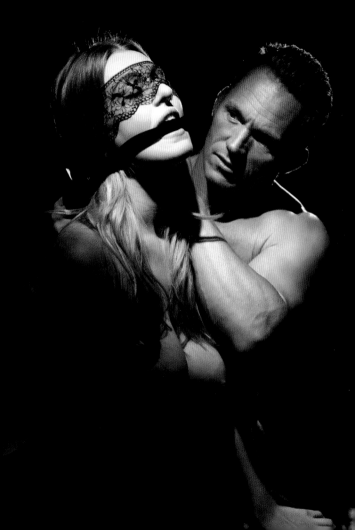

31 · Silent Night

GREAT SEX INVOLVES THE MIND at least as much as it involves the body, and a little psychology can go a long way when it comes to speeding orgasm. Many people assume that they have to make noise during sex to show their lover their appreciation. However, banning each other from making a single noise during sex can add a frisson on multiple levels.

First, we naturally want to do things that we can't, and denying that urge can give a delicious tease to those with any submissive streak: fighting the desperate need to groan as your lover does something particularly delicious. And second, it helps you focus attention on your lover as, without his or her vocalizations to steer you, you need to rely on his or her body language alone.

Signs that may indicate your partner is enjoying him- or herself include faster breathing, a flushed face and/or chest, and tensed muscles. Biting the lip and contorting the face into unusual expressions is common, too. As they near orgasm, they may move faster.

If you want to add more of a BDSM (bondage, discipline, dominance/ submission, and sadomasochism) element to proceedings, you could add a blindfold and gag to the encounter. You may decide that one of you is in a submissive role and the other in a dominant role, or you might decide to both wear gags in mutual torment. How you play is up to you, as long as you remember that you're not allowed to utter a single word until you come.

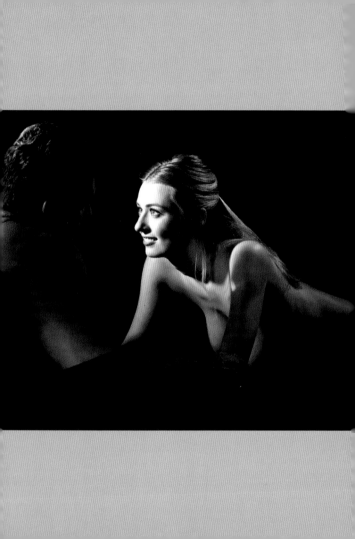

32 · Vampire Kisses

IF YOUR LOVER FINDS ORAL SEX too delicate to do the job, opt for a session of Vampire Kisses instead. Don't be too alarmed by the name—there's not going to be any biting. However, there will be a long, slow, steady suction designed to make your nerves tingle and set your senses alight.

This technique is not designed for people with sensitive nether regions: if you find yourself pulling away from overly enthusiastic caresses on a regular basis, it's better to opt for one of the gentler techniques. However, if you're a woman who has a lack of clitoral sensitivity or a man who finds he has issues with numbness or lack of sensation, then the extra stimulation could be just what you need.

Start by gently nibbling and sucking your way over your lover's skin, from neck to nethers. Once the clitoris or penis is erect, suck it into your mouth, gradually sucking harder based on your lover's response. Don't suck in too fast—but do keep the suction slow and steady.

Let your lips enclose the penis or clitoris and alternate suction with gentle breathing all over the area. The change in sensation will help your redoubled suction efforts feel all the more intense.

As your partner nears climax, you may want to add fingers or a toy to the equation too. Alternatively, you may find that the blend of intense suction and seductive breathing could send him or her over the edge all on its own.

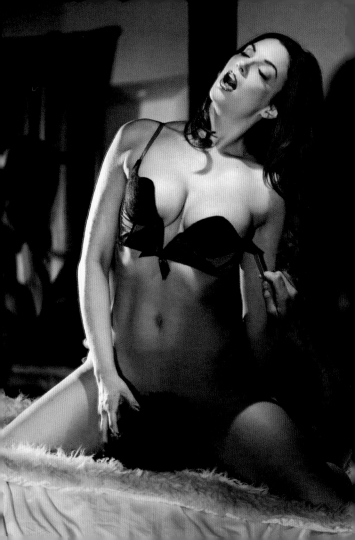

33 · In for the Night

EVERYONE HAS MOMENTS when they want to be selfish, and there's nothing wrong with demanding some solo satisfaction on occasion. In for the Night is designed for times when the woman's feeling frisky and the man isn't up for the challenge. However, all he needs to do to indulge his lover is lie back with his mouth open and his tongue stuck out, ready for action.

The woman then straddles the man's face, riding his tongue to spur her orgasm. She may choose to grind up against his nose or chin. She might choose to pull away so that he can only reach her with the very tip of his tongue. Or she might ask him to hold his tongue out flat, so that she can rub her clitoris over it in long, smooth strokes.

Not only does this help make orgasm super speedy by putting the woman in control of her own pleasure, but it can also help men learn more about their lover's desired cunnilingus technique. After all, if you don't have anything to do but lie there with your tongue sticking out, there's plenty of scope for your brain to take notes. In addition, men who have submissive fantasies or desires may find that this technique gives exactly the kind of thrill they need, and women with a dominant streak will be equally satisfied.

Alternatively, if the man is feeling up for a little more involvement, he can caress his lover's breasts as she rides his face, spank her buttocks, stroke and massage her back, or add one or more fingers to her vagina, anus, or both. However, it's best to let the woman lead the way. All too often, women feel embarrassed to admit their real desires, but if she's given a man to do with as she will, it's easy to learn what really drives her wild.

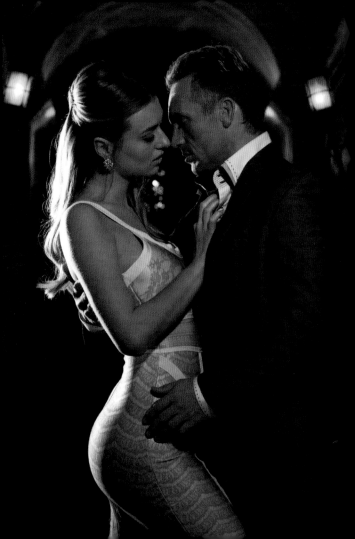

34 · Dirty Dancing

YOU DON'T HAVE TO TAKE YOUR CLOTHES OFF to have a good time. Instead, if you're overcome with passion when you're on a night out with your lover and you don't have time to drag each other home for a ravishing, opt for some Dirty Dancing instead. Extremely dirty dancing.

Go onto the dance floor with your lover, picking somewhere crowded enough that there won't be anything suspicious about getting super close. (No matter how crowded it is, don't even consider trying this at a wedding—you don't want to outshine the bride and groom with your passion.) Start slow dancing but instead of simply swaying from side to side, the woman should slide her thigh between her lover's and the pair of you should start grinding together.

Let the woman set the pace, as there's a much higher chance of her reaching climax than the man. Hold hands so that she can lean back or come close as she sees fit, and work some face stroking into your moves so it looks like you're simply having a romantic time. Relish the sensation of engorged clit rubbing against erect penis and let yourself get carried away with the music. If possible, stay on the dance floor until the woman has managed to grind her way to orgasm against the man. You may want to follow this with some Bathroom Bliss (#30) to sate the man's tension too.

If grinding alone doesn't do it for you, you can also get remote controlled toys for both men and women that send vibrations through your nether regions at a click of a controller key ring. Just make sure you don't lose the key ring—you don't want a stranger getting hold of it and inadvertently driving your lover wild with desire. Unless, of course, that's a fantasy the pair of you happen to share.

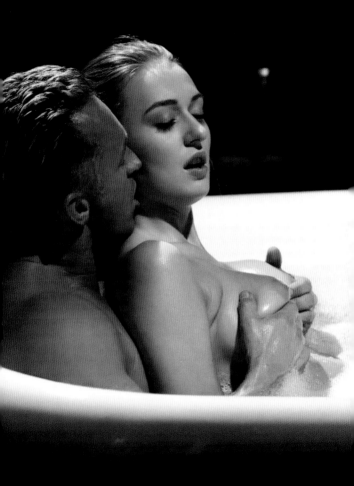

35 · Stress Relief

STRESS IS ONE OF THE MOST COMMON LIBIDO KILLERS, so what could be better than a sex act that releases tension for both of you? She gets to enjoy a sensual stroking, and he gets to enjoy fifteen minutes caressing his lover's breasts: talk about a mutually beneficial experience.

The breasts can be a wonderful erogenous zone. However, some women find their breasts get sensitive at certain times of the month, or even throughout the month. This doesn't mean breast massage is out: in fact, quite the opposite. Regular breast massage is thought to help improve breast sensitivity, turning pain into pleasure–or at least comfort.

Breast massage is great in the bath or shower as soap allows your hands to glide over your lover's skin easily, making it less likely you'll inadvertently give an uncomfortable squeeze. There's also the added bonus that soapy skin feels great underneath your fingertips.

Alternatively, use oil to make your hands glide over your lover's skin more smoothly. Start at the outer edges of the breast and slowly circle your fingertips inward, stopping just short of the nipple to build your lover's anticipation. Circle the breasts thirty times to the left then thirty times to the right using smooth strokes, only then moving your attention to the nipples.

For an added bit of kinky fun, once your time is almost up, the woman can start masturbating as the man masturbates over her breasts. Alternatively, she can stroke him and let him finish between her breasts. And of course, having thoroughly relaxed his lover's breasts, the man can always relax her nether regions with a stress relieving device. What could be more relaxing than orgasms all around?

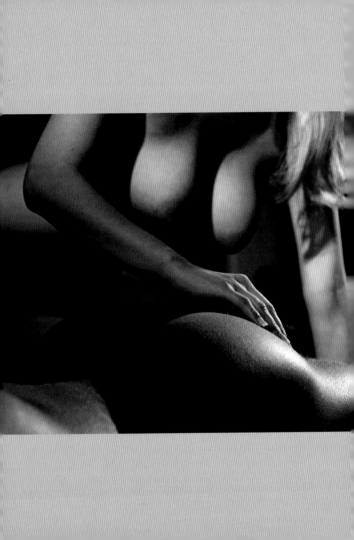

36 · Prostate with Pleasure

THE PROSTATE is a controversial body part. Some men find that a finger or two on the prostate can act as a near instant orgasm inducer. Others find the mere idea to be a total turn-off. Some people are open minded about the concept but would rather keep it as something for solo play rather than partnered sex. And then there are those who are up for giving it a go but aren't sure what to expect.

This is definitely something to check beforehand. No one wants an uninvited finger where the sun doesn't shine.

However, if your partner is willing, lube and latex gloves are your friends. Wear the latter both for safe sex and to help avoid your nails scratching your partner. Cover your finger(s) and your lover's anus liberally in oil or silicone-based lube, then slowly circle the anus until it starts to relax and you can push forward. Slide your finger in slowly and, as your finger gets deeper inside (two inches or more), feel around for a walnut-shaped lump on the upper wall of the anus. This is the prostate. Press it lightly, and circle your fingertip around it to see what elicits the most positive response. Some men like it if you press firmly into the prostate, while others prefer a lighter touch.

Some men prefer external prostate stimulation, through pressing against the perineum (the area between the balls and the anus) rather than inserting your finger into the anus. Although less instantly effective, it's much easier and doesn't require any specialist lubes or toys: just press that perineum as you work your man's shaft, and chances are, he'll have a smile on his face.

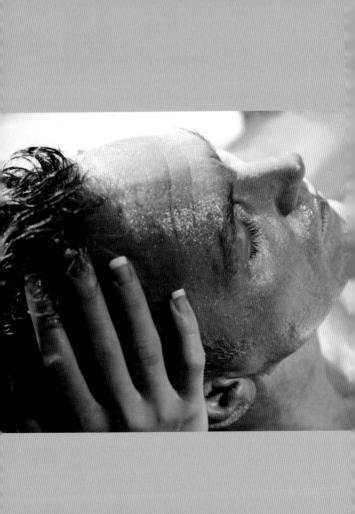

37 · Bath then Bed

WHAT COULD BE A BETTER WAY to end the day than with a sensual bath then bed? It's an easy way to make the most of your limited time–and, better yet, sharing a bath is good for the planet. Even ten minutes bathing each other can be bonding and relaxing, but if you can spare any more time, so much the better.

Soap each other all over, excluding the genital region, as soap can cause irritation. Use the suds to help your hands glide over each other's bodies and vary your caresses from soft strokes to more massaging grips. Pay attention to your lover's response and use the knowledge to refine your mental "body blueprint" of your partner.

Once you've thoroughly washed each other, dry each other with the warm towels and retire to the bedroom. As you've neglected your lover's nether regions because of the soap, now's time to redress the balance with some genital massage.

Use lube (not oil) to cover your hands, then explore your lover's genitals in intimate detail. When massaging a woman, try tracing your fingers up and down each side of the labia, rubbing the pubic mound, softly squeezing the clitoral shaft, and tapping the pads of the fingers across the whole genital region. For a man, try massaging the perineum (the area between the base of the penis and the anus), stroking just the shaft, sliding your fingers around the glans (aka head) of the penis, and softly stroking the balls. Whether you take things to conclusion with your hands or move to penetrative sex is entirely up to you.

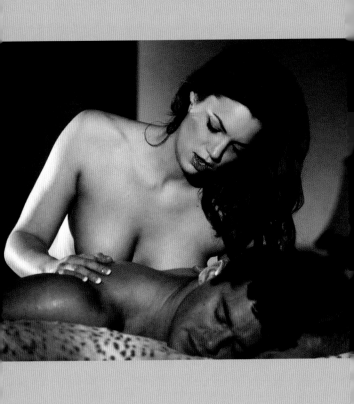

38 · Sleeping Like a Log

TAKE A TIP FROM THAI MASSAGE by using your entire body to caress your partner. The receiving partner lies flat on his or her front on the bed. The giving partner then covers his or her lover in lubricant or massage oil before lying on the receiver's back and wriggling against his or her skin.

If the woman is the giving partner, she can grind her pubic mound and clitoris against her lover as her breasts rub against his back. If the man is the giving partner, he can slide his penis in between her buttocks and stimulate himself between her cheeks.

You can also whisper sweet and dirty nothings in your lover's ear as you wriggle against him or her, to add extra heat and speed your mutual climax. Remember to talk slowly and softly and use silence on occasion so that your lover has to fill in the gaps in his or her own naughty imagination.

The giving partner should use his or her hands to caress his or her lover's shoulders and torso, and can also slide a hand underneath the receiver to give more direct stimulation. You can also incorporate toys into this, from a vibrating bullet underneath the receiving woman's clit to strap on sex teamed with grinding and wriggling if the woman is the giver.

As a slippery twist, put plastic sheets on the bed and use a mixture of bubble bath and oil with a few splashes of water so that your grinding results in lots of soap bubbles. However, do be careful not to get it anywhere intimate, as soaps can cause irritation, and finish off in the shower so you end up squeaky clean after getting dirty together.

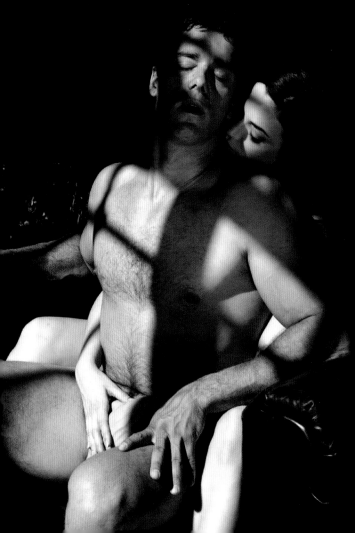

39 · Stroke of Midnight

FOR A NEW TWIST on the hand job that should get the job done in record time, try the Stroke of Midnight. Start by sitting behind your lover with your arms around his waist. Now, apply a generous measure of lubricant to your palms and put your hands together, palm to palm. Lattice your fingers together, raising both middle fingers so that they are sticking up while all your other fingers remain together.

Now, slot your hands over your lover's member, entering through the gap at the base of your palms. Let your middle fingers extend up the length of the penis and pulse your palms in and out as you slide your hands up and down the shaft. Your fingers will stimulate the sensitive frenulum (the string of flesh that connects the head of the penis to the shaft) while the pulsing of your hands mimics the muscular clenches of the vagina.

Try running your middle fingers from side to side as your hands pump up and down to see if you can find any super sensitive spots. For added intimacy, lean into your lover's body and kiss his neck or whisper naughty words in his ear.

For extra stimulation, this move can be teamed with strap-on sex. Simply change position so the man is sitting on the woman's lap on a chair. That way, he can guide the strap-on in and control the depth of penetration while she works wonders on his penis.

Alternatively, you can sandwich a vibrator between the man's back and buttocks and the woman's body. That way, she can grind her way to orgasmic bliss at the Stroke of Midnight.

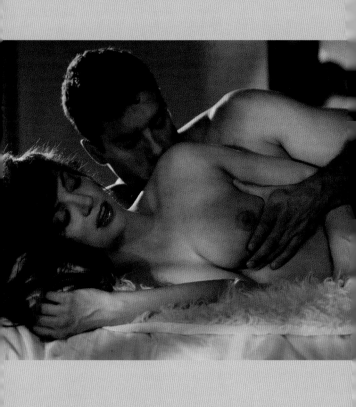

40 · Sweet Dreams

WHAT COULD BE BETTER than a bedtime story when you're drifting off to sleep? An erotic bedtime story, of course. All too many people rely on the physical alone to give their partner pleasure, but if you engage the mind as well as the body, you're a lot more likely to speed your lover's climax.

Women are thought to be particularly susceptible to erotic conversation. As such, help her drift off to sleep in sensual bliss by spooning her as you let your words work wonders. Cup her mons with one hand and encourage her to rock against it, using her body to indicate when your words are hitting the right spot.

As your lover nears orgasm, she may want you to continue talking dirty, or take over herself, leading the dirty talk in a direction she knows is a sure fire orgasm inducer. She might want silence so that she can focus on the physical sensations or the fantasies swimming through her mind. Pay as much attention to the way that her body moves as the words that she uses.

Continue until your lover reaches climax, then snuggle up and go to sleep. Alternatively, if you're feeling heated and both want to continue, swap positions so that the woman is spooning the man, working his shaft and trailing her fingertips over his balls as she whispers erotic inspirations in his ear.

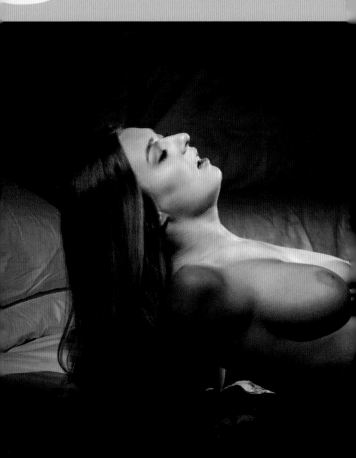

in Bangkok

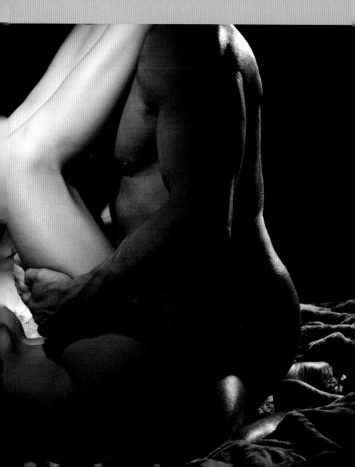

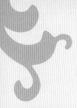

41 · One Night in Bangkok

QUICKIES HAVE THE REPUTATION for being hard and fast and, although this isn't always required, on occasion it can be just what the doctor ordered. Hard, fast sex can have an animal quality, raw and passionate. Some women find it can be painful, particularly if they have a sensitive cervix. This is why foreplay is essential before you have deep sex. Use a toy for speedy arousal, or opt for cunnilingus if your lover isn't into a battery-operated buzz.

Once the woman is feeling super-aroused, she should put one or more pillows underneath her hips. This angles her pelvis upward, making deep penetration easier for the man (meanwhile, the foreplay will have helped her cervix tilt back, keeping it out of the direct firing line once the man starts thrusting in earnest). The man lies on top of the woman who then raises her ankles to rest on his shoulders.

Now, it's simply a case of thrusting. Don't go for a deep stroke first off. Start with a few super shallow strokes, making her want more. Pull out on occasion and rub the head of your penis over her clit. Gauge her response by her wetness and moans, and make her wait just a fraction longer than she wants to before you start thrusting away. Continuing the foreplay during sex will help you both enjoy yourselves much more.

Once she's writhing in bliss, it's time to pull out the big guns. Start pounding, but keep an eye on her face so you can spot any discomfort. If it feels too deep, she can lower her feet onto the bed or remove the pillows from under her hips.

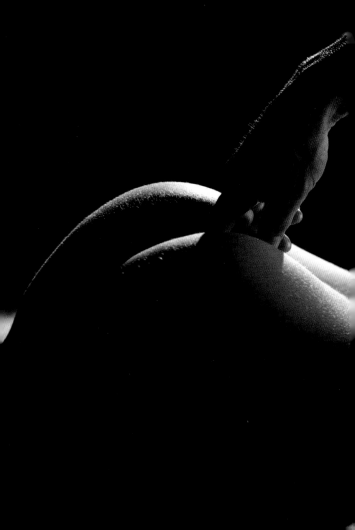

42 · Cocktail Time

IF YOU WANT FASTER CLIMAX THROUGH SEX, adding extra levels of stimulation will set you on the right path. Rather than focusing attention on just one erogenous zone, using a combination can help overwhelm the senses and lead to orgasmic bliss.

Although many women are reticent about anal sex, more are open to milder levels of anal play, such as fingering. The anus is packed with nerve endings and this, adding to the taboo nature of anal play, can help provide extra levels of pleasure to sex.

Start with the woman on all fours and the man kneeling behind her doggie style. Rather than going straight for penetration, start with some external anal play. Circle a latex-gloved and well-lubricated finger around the anus, waiting until you feel it start to relax at your touch prior to sliding it inside your lover. Add more lube if need be–better to have too much than not enough–and move slowly. Your lover can always push back if she wants it deeper, whereas overly fast anal penetration can be painful, or even cause tears to the anus (though using gloves helps reduce this risk).

Slide your finger in and out of the anus or, if that's too painful for your lover, try simply moving your finger around inside the anus. It's far more spacious inside than at the entrance, so many women find this more comfortable.

Once you're both ready, introduce the penis to the vagina, sliding it in slowly while your finger still works its magic in the woman's anus. You can alternate finger and penis thrusts or synchronise the two–all the better for her to imagine three-way action. Add more lube as required and keep the dual stimulation going until you both reach climax, unless requested otherwise.

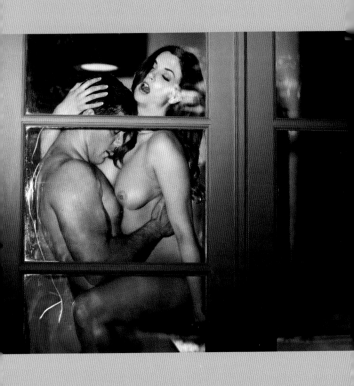

43 · Window (Un)Dressing

EXHIBITIONISM IS A COMMON fantasy, and you don't even have to leave the house to indulge your desires. Simply pull the sofa up to the window, then close the curtains or leave them as open as you dare, and get into position. Having sex while looking out the window, and seeing the world oblivious to you outside, can add an extra frisson to sex.

Window (Un)Dressing is easy: the man sits in the middle of the sofa, and the woman straddles him. You don't need to remove all your clothes—the woman simply needs to slip off her panties if she's wearing a skirt, or push down her pants if need be. Meanwhile, the man just has to undo his fly and push his trousers and underwear down to his knees. Leaving clothes on during sex can be hot—and as the session continues, pulling at each other's clothes to reveal more flesh can add extra heat.

The woman can alternate leaning forward to grind her clitoris against the base of her lover's shaft and/or his pubic area with more vigorous bouncing to provide stimulation through deep penetration. If she likes G-spot stimulation, she can lean back to better angle the head of the penis toward the G-spot.

Meanwhile, the man can use his hands to caress his lover's body through her clothes, or slide them underneath her top to stroke her skin and breasts. How you play it is up to you, but it's probably best to avoid leaning out of the window.

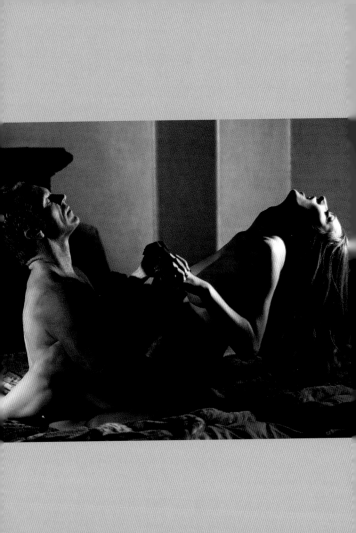

44 · Rock-a-Bye-Baby

ALTHOUGH THE NAME SOUNDS soothing, this position does take a little work for both of you, so it's not one for a night when you're looking for a lazy, indulgent session. However, it is incredibly intimate and allows both of you lots of scope for stimulation.

To get into position, sit in the middle of the bed facing each other, with your legs spread and backs to the bed head and foot accordingly. The woman then slides her legs over the top of her lover's, moving forward until she can slide him inside her, and wraps her legs around his waist. The man crosses his legs behind his partner's back. Then both lovers join hands and lean back, then forward, rocking against each other. This keeps the clitoris in almost constant contact with the man's pubic mound, meaning she's more likely to get the stimulation she needs to reach climax. She can also flex and pulse her Kegel muscles to increase sensation for both her and her lover.

One of the advantages of this position is that you can kiss throughout. It also allows plenty of scope for Tantric techniques, such as eye gazing and breathing each other's breath.

A cock ring can be added to this position to increase your chances of mutual climax. Opt for one with a vibrating bullet or, if you find vibrations too intense, simply choose one with a non-vibrating stimulator. Anything that increases stimulation of the clitoris is likely to serve you well when you want fast mutual pleasure.

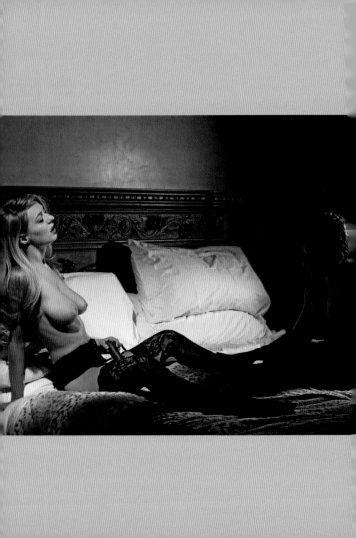

45 · Open Wide

IF YOU WANT TO make a man come in record time, giving him great visuals to enjoy along with hot sex is likely to reap rewards. Although it's often falsely claimed that women don't get visually aroused–in reality, they get physically aroused by a more diverse array of adult material than men–it's certainly true to say that, for the majority of men, a sexy view leads to sexual desire.

She kneels on the bed and spreads her legs as wide as possible to give her lover an X-rated view. For added kink, she can use a vibrator as her lover looks on. There's a reason that masturbation scenes are so popular in porn, and it'll get her ready for the hot and heavy action that's about to follow.

Once the woman feels sufficiently aroused, she adds an extra level of visual provocation by putting her hands on her buttocks and spreading them, to give her lover a graphic display of her most intimate parts. He can then start by worshipping her with his tongue to ensure she's definitely wet enough, then slide inside her. Start with a few shallow thrusts then gradually get deeper: by parting her buttocks, the woman will allow the deepest possible entry.

If that's still not enough for you and you both want a really intensely deep experience, the man can raise the woman's legs and tuck them under his arms while his partner holds her cheeks apart. He can then thrust his full length all the way inside her. Porntastic but super fast.

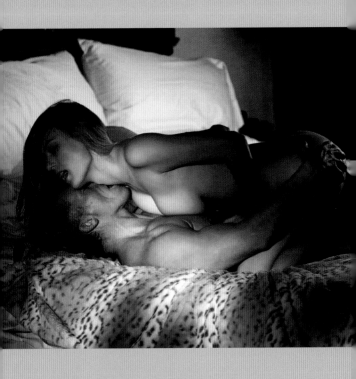

46 · CAT Nap

COITAL ALIGNMENT TECHNIQUE—better known as CAT—is a position that some studies claim increase women's chance of climax by up to 70 percent. It is like missionary but, rather than having his hips between his partner's thighs, the man shuffles upward once he's inside the woman so that the base of the shaft rubs against her clitoris. Rather than thrusting, he rocks and grinds and his partner does the same for much more clitoral stimulation.

This flipped version of the position is ideal for when the woman is feeling frisky and her partner is lacking in energy. To get into the CAT Nap position, the man lies on his back with his legs together and penis erect. The woman then straddles him to insert his penis into the vagina before lying flat on top of him, facing him. She then grinds away, using the base of his shaft to rub against her clit and flexes her Kegel muscles around him to increase blood flow to the area.

For a sexy twist on the CAT Nap, you can team it with One Night in Bangkok (#41) and cover your lover's chest in lubricant before you get into position. This will allow your bodies to slide against each other deliciously, offering a different sensation to usual sex. However, don't use oil for this unless you've both been tested for STIs and have pregnancy prevention in place as, unlike condom-safe lubricants, it can cause latex condoms to break.

Once she's had her fun, the woman can speed her movements and change to a thrusting motion to help her lover come, if the grinding hasn't offered him enough stimulation. Alternatively, you can flip position into missionary and the man can take control.

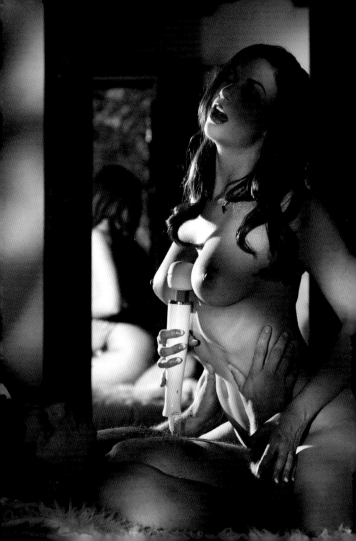

47 · Bedtime Buddies

FEELING FRISKY BUT DON'T HAVE TIME for an extended session? That's where a toy chest comes in very handy indeed. There's no need to use one toy at a time. Instead, take a plethora of bedtime buddies with you: in the fight for more mutual orgasms, see your toy stash as the allies that will help you get exactly what you need.

Start by taking one cock ring with dual stimulators: one for his perineum and one for her clit. Slide it onto the man's erect member, checking that the clitoral stimulator is in the right position. Add a small butt plug to massage the man's prostate. He should insert it with lots of lube to ensure it's quick and easy, but comfortable. If the woman is also into anal play, there's nothing to stop her from inserting a plug too. (Get his and hers plugs so that you don't get them mixed up, and clean thoroughly after use as you can transmit infections through toys as well as exchanging fluids directly.)

Now, throw in a hand held wand-style vibe for the woman, and you're sure to rev each other's engines in record time. Be warned, wand style vibrators are not for the faint hearted as they pack an incredibly powerful buzz. However, this does make them ideal if you struggle to reach climax in any other way. (The head of the wand can also be used on a man's perineum to pleasurable effect if he's into vibrations.)

The best position to get everything involved at once? The man sits on a chair, the woman straddles him with her clit on the vibrating stimulator, and the man wraps his arms around her waist to hold her in position, leaving her hands free to use the magic wand on her breasts, clitoral shaft or, by reaching behind herself, his thighs and balls.

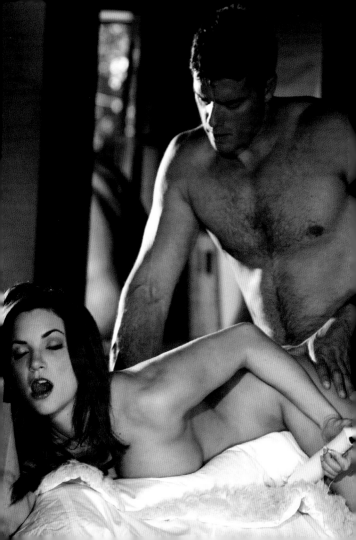

48 · Pillow Talk

PILLOWS CAN BE A GIRL'S BEST FRIEND. Many women have fond memories of early sexual experiences, grinding against a pillow or similar, but as time goes on, it can be easy to forget the simple bliss of pressing the pudenda against a soft but firm surface, and instead rely on penetration to get your kicks. However, if you want fast pleasure, it's time to raid those memory banks and use anything you can that increases your chances of orgasm.

A pillow can be taken to a whole other level of pleasure if teamed with a magic wand style vibrator: a powerful toy that is noisy enough to leave you in no doubt as to the power it packs. Many women find wands thrilling but too intense, particularly on the higher levels. However, by putting a pillow between the woman and the toy, it softens the vibrations, and the pillow gives extra surface area to grind against. Turn the vibrator up and down until you find the perfect level of vibration through the pillow for you.

To enjoy Pillow Talk, the woman should lie face down on the pillow, holding the toy underneath it in the desired position, and grind against it as she desires. Her partner then simply has to slide into her from behind, giving (and getting) deep penetration to team with the clitoral thrills. He can caress her breasts, kiss her neck, whisper erotic ideas in her ear, and let his hands play over her body as the pillow and wand work their magic down below. Similarly, the woman can use her hands to control the vibrator, caress her breasts, or, if she reaches behind herself, play with her lover's balls.

Just what you need to set you up for sweet dreams and a satisfying slumber after a long, hard day.

Brimming with creative inspiration, how-to projects, and useful information to enrich your everyday life, Quarto Knows is a favorite destination for those pursuing their interests and passions. Visit our site and dig deeper with our books into your area of interest: Quarto Creates, Quarto Cooks, Quarto Homes, Quarto Lives, Quarto Drives, Quarto Explores, Quarto Gifts, or Quarto Kids.

First published in 2015 by Quiver,
an imprint of The Quarto Group,
100 Cummings Center, Suite 265-D,
Beverly, MA 01915, USA.
T (978) 282-9590 F (978) 283-2742
www.QuartoKnows.com

Quiver titles are also available at discount for retail, wholesale, promotional, and bulk purchase. For details, contact the Special Sales Manager by email at specialsales@quarto.com or by mail at The Quarto Group, Attn: Special Sales Manager, 401 Second Avenue North, Suite 310, Minneapolis, MN 55401 USA.

19 18   4 5

ISBN: 978-59233-667-8

Cover design by traffic
Photography by Holly Randall

Printed and bound in Hong Kong